BE WELL AGAIN

(Herbal Remedies for Ailments)

**Dr. Isabella Morales
& Dr. Rajesh Patel**

Be Well Again:

Herbal Remedies for Ailments

Copyright © 2023 by Dr. Isabella Morales
and Dr. Rajesh Patel

Table of Contents

Introduction to Herbal Healing

In our present day society, where modern medicine typically takes stage in the healthcare landscape, we still hold an appreciation for the ancient practice of herbal healing. The utilization of plants and herbs for medicinal purposes has been a part of human culture for thousands of years. Today it remains highly valued and effective as an approach to promoting health and well-being. In this chapter we embark on a captivating journey, into the realm of herbal healing delving into its history, the core principles that underpin it and the enduring reasons why it has stood the test of time.

The Timeless Wisdom of Herbal Healing

Herbal healing also known as herbalism or phytotherapy involves the utilization of plants, herbs and botanical substances, for therapeutic purposes. This practice has been a part of civilization since ancient times. Various ancient civilizations such as the Egyptians, Greeks, Chinese and Indigenous peoples across continents have relied on the healing properties of plants to address a wide range of ailments.

What distinguishes healing is its connection to nature. It adopts an approach that acknowledges the interplay between humans and their environment while emphasizing the significance of balance and harmony. Herbs are not merely viewed as remedies for symptoms. Rather as tools for achieving overall well-being.

The Rise of Modern Medicine

Although herbalism boasts a history, the emergence of modern medicine in the 19th and 20th centuries brought significant changes to healthcare practices. The discovery of antibiotics and advancements in drugs revolutionized the treatment of diseases and many chronic conditions. Consequently herbal remedies took a backseat over time leading to their decline, in parts of the world.

Modern medicine undoubtedly yielded outcomes; however it also had its limitations. The focus on treating symptoms rather than addressing root causes, along with the potential for side effects left some people seeking alternatives. Even alongside its high cost. This change in viewpoint has sparked a renewed interest in herbal remedies.

The Return to Natural Remedies

In years there has been a growing awareness of the limitations and potential drawbacks of relying on pharmaceutical drugs. Many individuals have started exploring alternative therapies leading to resurgence, in herbal healing.

One of the reasons behind this renewed interest is a desire for natural and holistic approaches to health. People are increasingly seeking treatments that take into account not physical symptoms but the mental, emotional and spiritual aspects of well-being. Herbalism aligns with this viewpoint acknowledging that health is multifaceted concept.

The Power of Plants

Plants are living organisms that have evolved over millions of years developing an array of chemical compounds to safeguard themselves from predators and environmental stressors. These inherent chemicals, commonly known as phytochemicals are precisely what make herbs valuable for medicinal purposes.

Herbs contain a range of phytochemicals with numerous properties. Some herbs possess inflammatory compounds while others boast antioxidants, antimicrobial agents or pain relieving components. The combination of these phytochemicals found in herbs offers an intricate approach to healing.

Holistic Healing

At the core of herbal healing lies the concept of holistic healing which recognizes the interconnectedness, between the mind, body and spirit.

This viewpoint emphasizes the significance of tackling the root causes of diseases rather than

just managing their symptoms. Herbalists
frequently collaborate with individuals to pinpoint
not just the symptoms they are encountering but
also the emotional and lifestyle aspects that could
be influencing their health problems. Through
the utilization of this approach herbal medicine
aims to rebalance and rejuvenate the individual as
a whole.

The Role of Herbalists

Herbalists are professionals who specialize in
using herbs, for healing purposes. They undergo
training to understand the characteristics of herbs
their interactions and how to create personalized
herbal remedies for individuals. Herbalists work
closely with their clients considering their unique
constitution, medical history and current health
concerns.

One of the advantages of herbalism is its
approach. Even if two individuals have the
ailment they may receive herbal remedies tailored
to their specific needs. This customized care is an
aspect of herbal healing that distinguishes it from
one size fits all approaches.

The Journey Ahead

As we delve deeper into the realm of herbal healing we will explore the captivating history of herbalism, gain knowledge about herb properties, learn how to prepare herbal remedies effectively and discover their applications, for various health concerns.

Herbal healing does not reject modern medicine. Rather complements it as an approach that can enhance our overall well-being. In the chapters that follow, we will embark on a journey of discovery and equip ourselves with valuable knowledge and skills to harness the healing potential of herbs while taking control of our own health.

Chapter One

Exploring the Origins of Herbal Medicine

The captivating story of medicine takes us on a journey through time highlighting humanity's enduring bond with the natural world and our relentless pursuit of well-being and healing. In this chapter we will delve into the tapestry of herbalism investigating its beginnings, development and the profound influence it has had on cultures worldwide.

Ancient Beginnings

The roots of medicine reach into the annals of human history. Archeological evidence suggests that our distant ancestors began utilizing plants for purposes far back as 60,000 years ago. These early remedies were likely a result of trial and error, observation of animals and an innate connection with the environment.

Civilizations from antiquity such as the Sumerians, Egyptians and Chinese meticulously documented their use of plants on clay tablets and papyrus scrolls. Among these records is the Ebers Papyrus dating back, to 1550 BCE—an invaluable medical text encompassing a treasure trove of herbal remedies employed by ancient Egyptians to address various ailments.

The Wisdom of the Greeks and Romans

The ancient civilizations of Greece and Rome played a role in advancing the field of medicine. Hippocrates, who is widely regarded as the "Father of Medicine", placed emphasis on the utilization of herbs for healing purposes. He firmly believed in the body's natural healing abilities and promoted an approach, to medical treatments.

During the first century CE Dioscorides, a physician, pharmacologist and botanist authored a renowned work known as "De Materia Medica." This remarkable piece of work documented the characteristics, uses and benefits of plants making it a trusted and authoritative source, for herbalists throughout many generations.

Herbal Medicine Traditions Across Different Continents

Throughout history diverse regions have independently developed their systems of medicine. Ayurveda in India, Traditional Chinese Medicine (TCM) American herbalism and African herbal traditions each have their methods of utilizing herbs for healing.

For instance Ayurveda takes an approach by considering an individual's constitution (dosha) when prescribing remedies. TCM also emphasizes restoring balance to the body's energy (qi) through herbs. Native American herbalism deeply relies on plant knowledge passed down through generations. Similarly African herbal traditions draw upon plant wisdom for medicinal purposes.

The Middle Ages and the Revival of Herbal Medicine

During Europe's middle Ages, monks and nuns in gardens played a role in preserving and advancing knowledge about herbal medicine. Influential figures like Hildegard of Bingen, a herbalist and mystic contributed insights into the healing properties of plants.

In the Renaissance period that followed there was a renewed interest, in exploring the potential of medicine.

Nicholas Culpeper, an herbalist, from England and Paracelsus a herbalist from Switzerland questioned methods and promoted the utilization of herbs for healing ailments. During the century Culpepers book titled "The Complete Herbal" gained popularity as a manual, for herbal remedies.

Herbal Medicine in Colonial America

When European settlers reached the Americas they encountered an abundance of plants and herbal practices. The influence of remedies, on early American herbalism was significant as people shared and adapted their knowledge of local plants. During the colonial era herbal texts like "Culpepers American Herbal" were published, incorporating indigenous herbs.

The Rise of Modern Medicine

The progress of medicine during the 20th centuries marked remarkable advancements driven by scientific discoveries, the development of pharmaceutical drugs and the establishment of rigorous medical practices. While these breakthroughs revolutionized healthcare and saved lives they also resulted in a decline in the utilization of herbal remedies across many regions worldwide.

However there has been resurgence in interest towards medicine as people seek more natural and holistic approaches to health. Herbalist's wisdom is being rediscovered as individuals recognize its value. Additionally scientific research has shed light on the properties of herbs providing validation for their effectiveness.

In today's world there is coexistence between herbalism and modern medicine. Healthcare practitioners increasingly acknowledge the importance of integrating remedies into treatment plans. Meanwhile individuals are turning to herbs for care and complementary therapies.

The continuation of tradition in medicine stands as a testament, to both plants enduring power and the wisdom passed down by our ancestors.

In this book we will delve into the world of healing taking inspiration from traditions and combining it with modern scientific knowledge. Together we will discover how herbs can enhance our well-being and promote a lifestyle, in today's world.

Chapter Two

Understanding Herbs and Their Characteristics

As we delve into the world of healing it becomes crucial to grasp the essence of this practice; the herbs themselves. Herbs are not merely plants, with foliage; they hold within them a wealth of compounds that can provide numerous benefits for our health and overall well-being. In this chapter we will explore the captivating realm of herbs their distinct properties and the factors that influence their effectiveness in promoting healing.

The Rich Diversity of Herbs

Herbs encompass a ranging and diverse collection of plants each possessing its unique set of characteristics. These plants can be grouped into categories encompassing herbs (those with strong scents), culinary herbs (used in cooking), medicinal herbs (valued for their healing properties) and ornamental herbs (cultivated for their aesthetic appeal).

In our journey we will primarily focus on herbs – those highly regarded for their effects. They can further be classified based on their healing actions, such, as inflammatory properties, antimicrobial abilities or calming qualities.

The Bioactive Compounds Found in Herbs

What sets herbs apart as formidable healers is the multitude of compounds they contain. These compounds have been formed over years of evolution as plants have developed chemical defenses to safeguard themselves against pests, diseases and the pressures of the environment. Phytochemicals refer to the chemicals in herbs that contribute to their therapeutic qualities. These encompass alkaloids, flavonoids, terpenes and essential oils, among substances. Each phytochemical serves a purpose in ensuring the survival of the plant. They can also contribute to our well-being when utilized appropriately.

Plant Parts and Their Uses

Herbs go beyond their leaves; they encompass a range of plant components. Common plant parts used in herbal remedies include:

Leaves; Leaves are often infused in teas due to their abundance in essential oils and antioxidants which offer numerous health benefits.

Roots; The grounding and tonifying properties of roots make them ingredients. They can be dried, powdered or tinctured for use in remedies.

Flowers; Flowers are not only beautiful. Flowers also contain essential oils and other beneficial compounds. They are frequently used in herbal teas and topical preparations

Seeds; Seeds possess both value and medicinal properties. They can be ground into powders and also for oil extraction.

Bark; Known for its astringent qualities, bark is commonly utilized to create decoctions or tinctures.

Each part of the plant serves purposes and herbalists carefully select the component based on the desired therapeutic effects.

The diversity within each herb category is significant because there are species and varieties. Consider mint as an example, where you'll find types like peppermint, spearmint and chocolate mint. Each type offers its flavor profile along, with distinct medicinal properties.

The selection of plant species and varieties is important because different plants can have varying levels of compounds. For instance peppermint *(Mentha × piperita)* is recognized for its menthol content, which adds to its cooling and calming effects. Recognizing these distinctions is vital when choosing the herbs for remedies.

The Significance of Plant Species and Varieties

In every category of herbs there exists a range of species and varieties. Let's consider the world of mint as an example. Mint encompasses species, like peppermint, spearmint and chocolate mint each possessing its flavor profile and medicinal qualities.

The selection of plant species and varieties holds importance because different plants may contain varying levels of compounds. For instance peppermint (Mentha × piperita) is renowned for its menthol content, which contributes to its cooling and soothing properties. Recognizing these distinctions becomes crucial when choosing the herbs for remedies.

Growing and Sourcing Herbs

Cultivation methods and sourcing play a role in determining the quality of herbs used in remedies. Many herbalists prefer to grow their herbs under conditions ensuring they remain free from pesticides and other contaminants.

Ethical harvesting practices such as wildcrafting are highly valued by herbalists. When conducted responsibly it aids in preserving native plant populations while also providing a source of herbs.

For individuals who lack access to herb, dried herbs serve as an alternative. Drying techniques allow for preservation while maintaining their potency and when stored correctly, they can last months or even years.

The Role of Terroir

Like wine the idea of terroir also applies to herbs. Terroir encompasses the factors such, as soil, climate and geography that impact the taste and overall quality of herbs. Different regions or types of soil can lead to variations, in the chemical composition and flavors of herbs, which ultimately affect their properties. When herbalists choose herbs they consider the concept of terroir as it plays a role in the effectiveness and taste of preparations.

To fully harness the healing capabilities of herbs, proper preparation is essential. There are methods for preparing herbs;

1. **Infusions;** this involves steeping herbs in water to make teas or infusions which works well for plant parts like leaves and flowers.

2. **Decoctions;** Root, bark and seed herbs are simmered in water to extract their compounds. Decoctions tend to be more potent than infusions.

3. **Tinctures;** Herbs are macerated in alcohol or glycerin to create extracts. Tinctures have a longer shelf life and are easy to measure out for dosage purposes.

4. **Salves and Ointments;** oils and extracts are combined with carriers like beeswax to produce remedies, for skin issues.

The choice of preparation method depends on the desired effect and the specific herb being used.

It's important to note that while herbs offer healing potential they also come with risks. Certain herbs may interact negatively with medications while others can have effects if used improperly or excessively. Therefore it is crucial to approach medicine with knowledge and caution.

As we explore further into the realm of remedies we will dive deeper into understanding the characteristics of herbs, their practical uses, for addressing various health issues and the proper methods to prepare and utilize them in a safe and beneficial manner.

Chapter Three

Herbal Recipes and Remedies for Common Cold and Flu

During the colder months we often find ourselves grappling with the common cold and flu. These viral infections can make us feel miserable with symptoms such as a runny nose, coughing, sore throat, congestion and fatigue. Herbal remedies can provide some relief by easing symptoms bolstering the immune system and promoting faster recovery. In this chapter we will explore a range of recipes and remedies that can assist in combating these illnesses.

Understanding the Common Cold and Flu

Before delving into solutions it is crucial to differentiate between the common cold and the flu. Although both are respiratory infections caused by viruses, they stem from different types of viruses and manifest certain distinct symptoms.

Common Cold; the common cold is typically brought on by rhinoviruses. Its hallmark symptoms include a congested nose, sneezing, coughing and a sore throat. Generally speaking it has a milder onset compared to the flu and tends to resolve quickly.

Influenza (Flu); the flu is caused by influenza viruses and tends to produce severe symptoms. These may encompass fever, body aches or pains, fatigue and a dry cough. The flu can also cause complications especially in people who are susceptible.

Herbal Teas, for Relieving Symptoms

When it comes to managing flu symptoms herbal teas offer a comforting and easily accessible solution. Here are a couple of tea recipes that may help alleviate your discomfort;

#Ginger and Lemon Tea;

Ginger is well known for its inflammatory properties and ability to boost the immune system. Adding some lemon provides a dose of vitamin C.

To make this tea, simply slice some ginger add it to a cup of hot water squeeze in the juice of half a lemon and sweeten with honey according to your taste.

#Peppermint and Eucalyptus Tea;

Peppermint can effectively relieve congestion while eucalyptus offers soothing benefits for the system.

For this tea steep a peppermint tea bag in water and add a drops of eucalyptus essential oil (make sure it's safe for consumption) to create a refreshing decongestant blend.

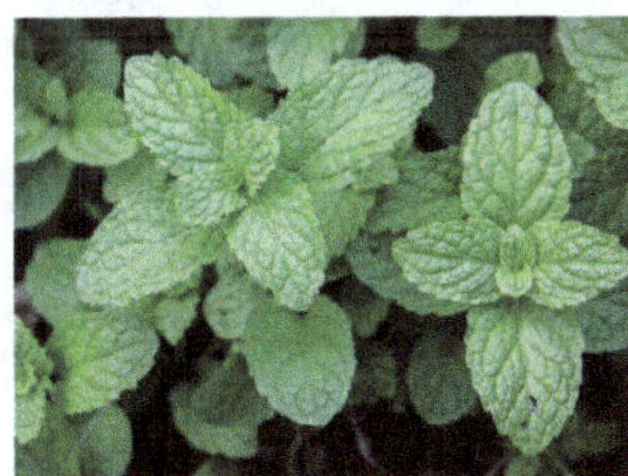

Peppermint Leaves

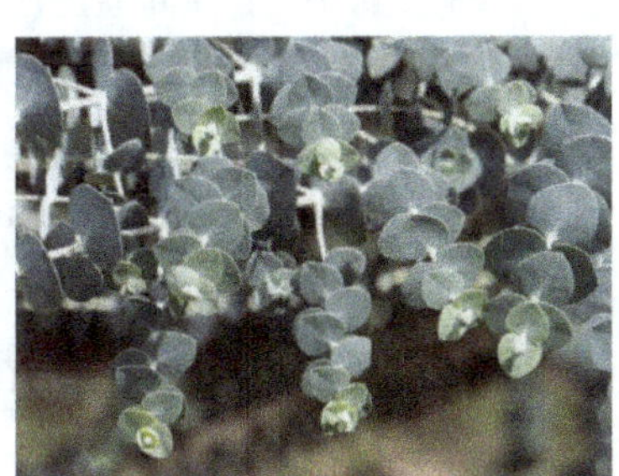

Eucalyptus Leaves

#Thyme and Honey Tea;

Thyme possesses properties that can help with coughs and sore throats.

To prepare this tea, steep either fresh or dried thyme leaves in water. Sweeten with honey as desired.

Herbal Steam Inhalation

Inhaling steam infused with herbs is a way to find relief from congestion while opening up your airways. Here's how you can do it;

1. **Eucalyptus Steam;**

Boil water, in a pot then add a drop of eucalyptus oil. Remove from heat.

Cover your head with a towel. Position yourself above the pot while inhaling the steam. Make sure to maintain a distance to prevent any burns.

Take slow breaths, for around 5-10 minutes in order to help clear your passages.

2. Steam with Herbal Blend;

Prepare a blend by combining dried herbs such, as chamomile, thyme and eucalyptus.

Bring water to a boil add the blend and allow it to steep for a minutes.

Inhale the steam as mentioned before.

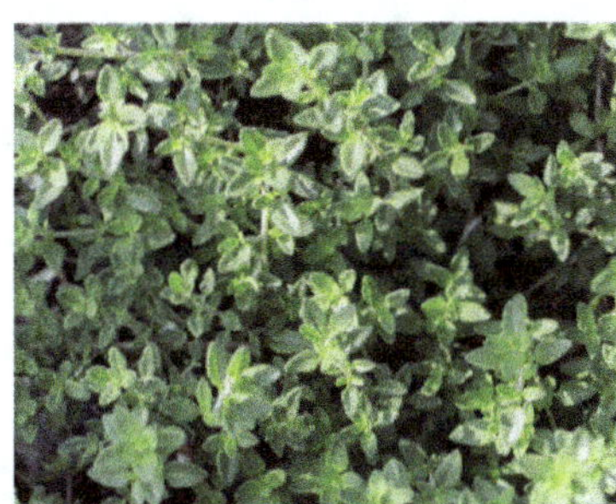

Thyme Leaves

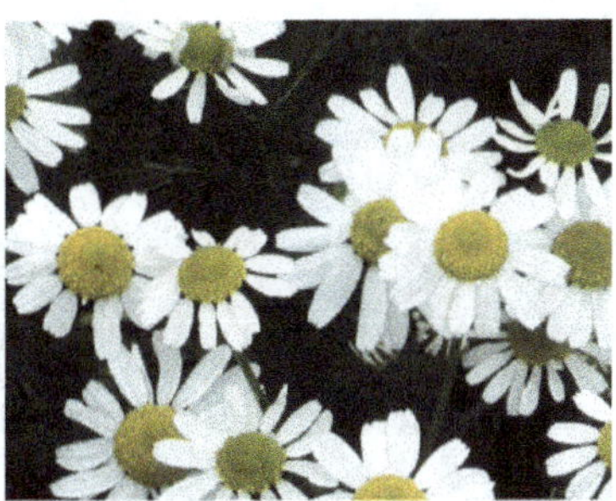

chamomile Leaves

Using Herbal teas to alleviate symptoms

When it comes to managing cold and flu symptoms herbal teas are a popular and comforting option. Here are some herbal tea recipes that may provide relief;

You can make your own herbal cough syrup using ingredients, which can provide relief without the additives often found in commercial syrups. Follow this recipe;

Ingredients;

- 1 cup of honey (preferably raw)
- 1 tablespoon of freshly grated ginger
- 1 tablespoon of dried thyme leaves
- Juice from 1 lemon

Instructions;

1. Gently warm the honey in a saucepan, over low heat. It's important not to boil it as you want to preserve its properties.
2. Add the ginger. Dried thyme leaves to the warm honey and stir well to combine.
3. Let the mixture simmer on heat for 5-10 minutes allowing the herbs to infuse into the syrup.
4. Remove the saucepan from heat, strain out the herbs and let the syrup cool down.
5. Once cooled add the lemon juice to the syrup. Mix thoroughly.

6. Store your cough syrup in a glass jar in
    your refrigerator and take 1- 2 teaspoons
    whenever needed for soothing coughs.

Immune-Boosting Herbal Tincture

Additionally it's essential to focus on building an immune system as it plays a crucial role, in preventing and combating colds and flu.

Here's a recipe, for a remedy that can help strengthen your system;

Ingredients;

1 part echinacea root (Echinacea purpurea)

1 part astragalus root (Astragalus membranaceus)

1/2 part elderberry (Sambucus nigra)

1/2 part ginger root (Zingiber officinale)

1 part alcohol (vodka or brandy)

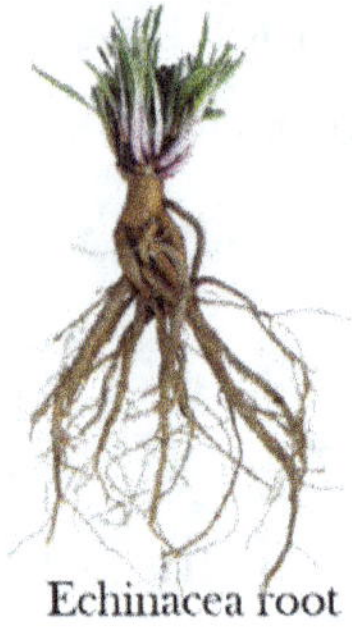

Echinacea root

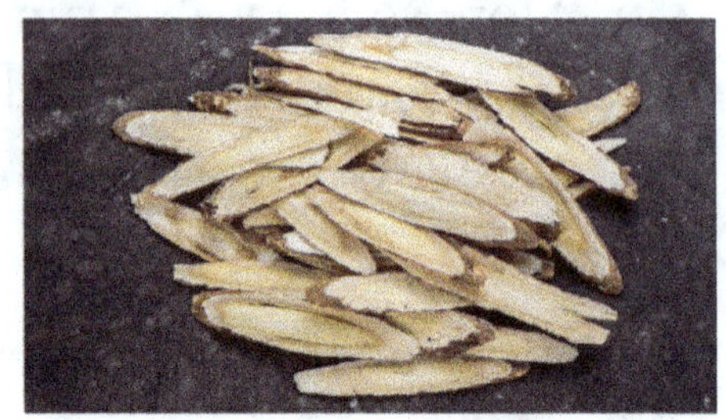

Astragalus root

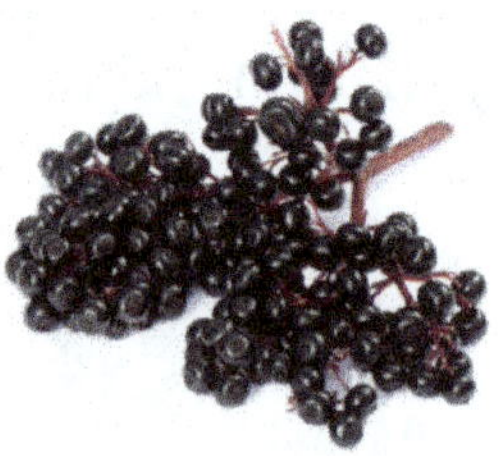

Elderberry

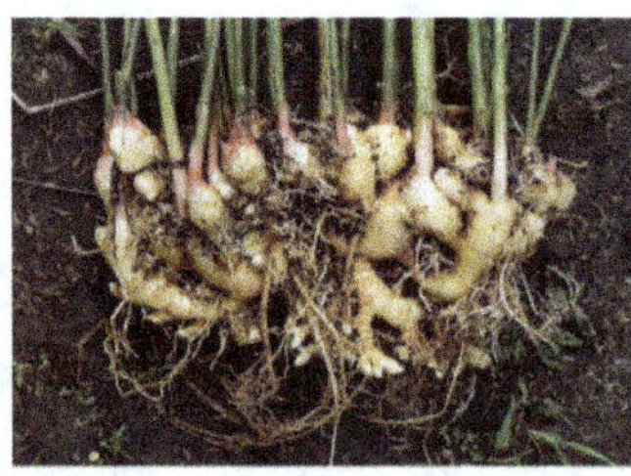

Ginger root

Instructions;

1. Get a glass jar. Combine the dried herbs.

2. Pour alcohol over the herbs making sure they are completely covered.

3. Seal the jar tightly. Give it a shake every day for about 4-6 weeks to allow the herbs to infuse.

4. Once the infusion period is over strain the tincture into a dark glass bottle.

How to Make Your Herbal Chest Rub

A homemade chest rub can provide relief from congestion and coughing. Here's a simple recipe;

Ingredients;

- 1/4 cup of coconut oil
- 10 drops of eucalyptus oil
- 10 drops of peppermint essential oil
- 5 drops of lavender essential oil

Instructions;

1. Take a bowl. Combine the solid coconut oil with the essential oils.
2. Mix everything thoroughly until all the ingredients are well blended.
3. Transfer the mixture into a container, with a lid.
4. Apply an amount to your chest and throat before bedtime. Whenever you need relief from congestion.

Importance of Rest and Hydration

Remember that getting rest and staying hydrated are elements for recovering from colds and flu. While herbal teas and remedies can alleviate symptoms it's equally important to allow your body time to heal. Ensure you drink plenty of fluids, get rest and pay attention to what your body needs.

These natural herbal recipes and remedies for colds and flu are intended to provide relief while supporting your body's healing processes.

While herbs can offer support during times of illness, it's crucial to seek guidance from a healthcare professional particularly if you have existing health conditions or are taking any medications. Herbal remedies can complement treatments. They should never be seen as a substitute for professional medical advice when necessary.

Chapter Four

Herbal Remedies for Stress and Anxiety

In our paced and frequently chaotic society stress and anxiety have emerged as widespread issues that affect our general state of wellness. In this chapter we will delve into the calming world of remedies, for managing stress and anxiety.

Understanding Stress and Anxiety

Before we explore remedies it's crucial to grasp the essence of stress and anxiety. Although they are experiences there are often areas of overlap;

Stress; Stress is the body's response to a perceived threat or demand whether real or imagined. It triggers a reaction known as the "fight or flight" response leading to alertness increased heart rate and other bodily changes.

Anxiety; Anxiety refers to a feeling of unease, fear or apprehension that often lacks a cause or identifiable threat. It can manifest as restlessness, irritability and physical symptoms such as muscle tension.

While occasional stress and anxiety are occurrences in life, chronic or excessive levels can have effects, on mental and physical well-being. This is where herbal remedies can provide support.

Herbal Adaptogens

Adaptogenic herbs belong to a category that assists the body in adapting to stress and maintaining equilibrium. They support the body's ability to respond to stressors while promoting a sense of tranquility. Some known adaptogens include;

Ashwagandha (Withania somnifera);
Ashwagandha is an herb renowned for its calming properties and its ability to reduce stress levels.

Rhodiola (Rhodiola rosea); It has the potential to regulate cortisol levels and induce a sense of relaxation. Rhodiola, scientifically known as

Rhodiola rosea is an adaptogen that boosts the body's ability to cope with stress. It is commonly used to combat tiredness and improve clarity.

Holy Basil, also referred to as Tulsi holds a place, in medicine due, to its soothing qualities. It can help reduce anxiety and promote emotional well-being.

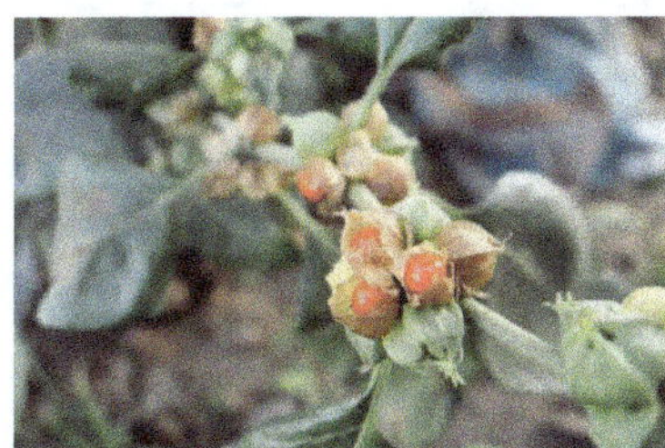

Ashwagandha

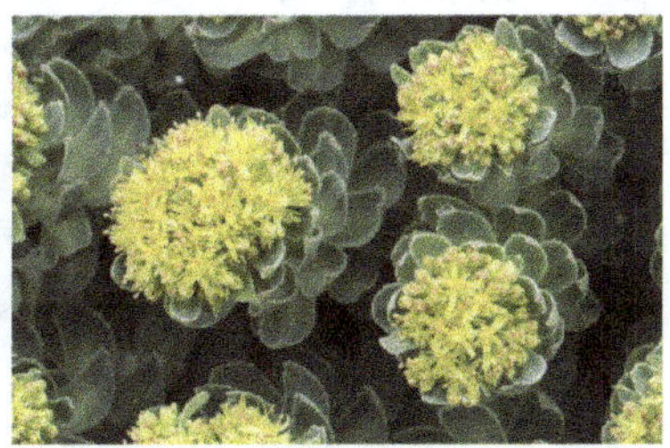

Rhodiola

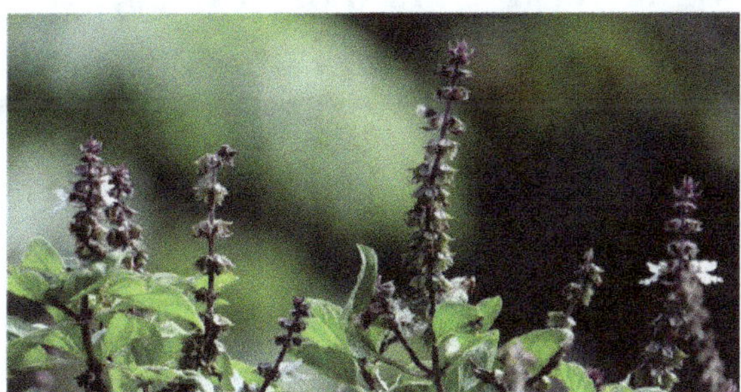

Holy Basil

Herbal Nervines

Nervine herbs fall into the category of herbs that provide support to the system helping to calm and soothe frayed nerves. There are a few noteworthy nervine herbs worth mentioning;

1. Lemon Balm (Melissa officinalis); Lemon balm is an herb that acts as a nervine bringing about an uplifting effect. It is often used to alleviate anxiety and improve mood.

2. Chamomile (Matricaria chamomilla); Chamomile is a known nervine herb recognized for its ability to promote relaxation and relieve tension. Many people enjoy it as a soothing tea.

3. Passionflower (Passiflora incarnata); Passionflower is known for its nervine properties that aid in reducing anxiety and enhancing sleep quality. It is frequently utilized in remedies targeting stress and insomnia.

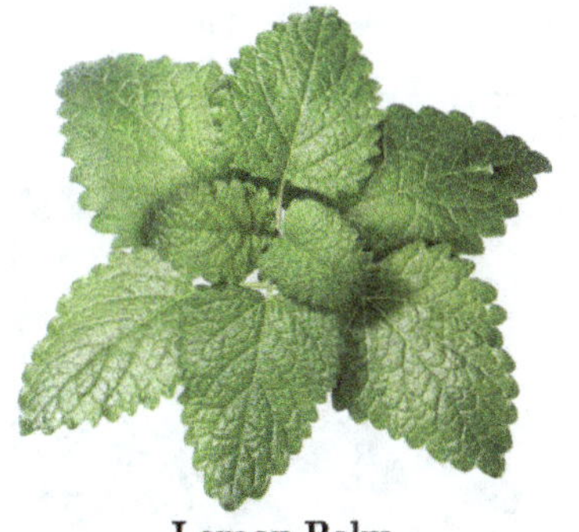

Lemon Balm

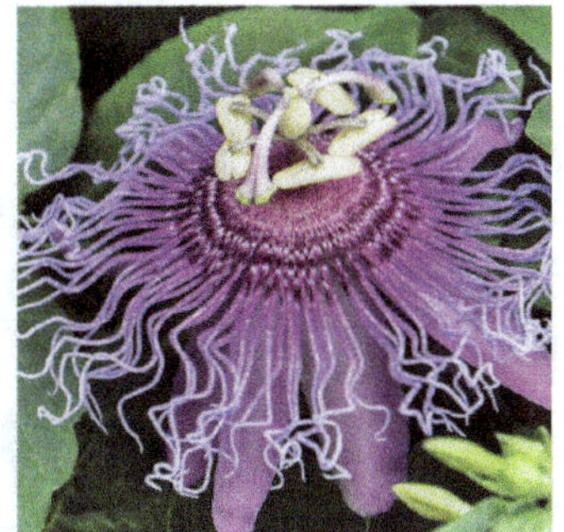

Passionflower

Within the realm of nervines there exists another subgroup called relaxant herbs, which possess calming effects, on the body. These are often employed to alleviate stress or anxiety. Let's explore some examples;

1. Valerian (Valeriana officinalis); Valerian is a relaxant renowned for its ability to induce relaxation and improve sleep quality. It finds usage in cases involving anxiety disorders or insomnia.

2. Kava Kava (Piper methysticum); Hailing from the South Pacific kava kava is an age herb known for its powerful relaxation inducing effects. Its

primary purpose revolves around reducing anxiety levels and fostering tranquility.

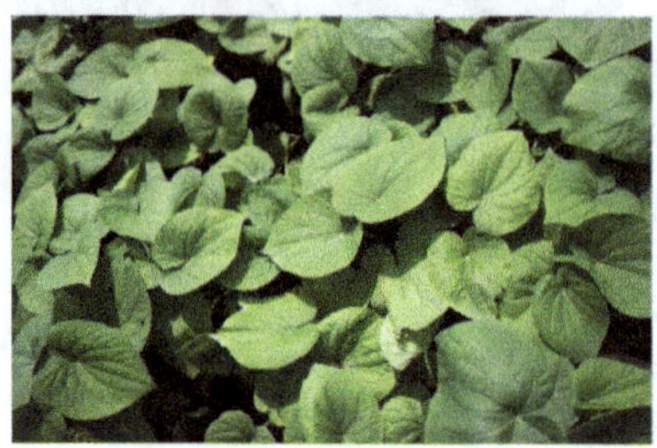

Kava Kava

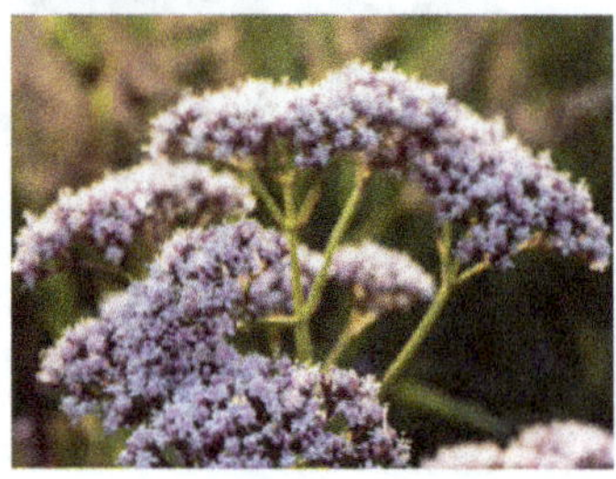

Valerian

Herbal Anxiolytics

There are herbs that have an effect on anxiety aiding in the relief of symptoms and promoting a feeling of tranquility. Some popular herbs known for their properties include;

Lavender (Lavandula angustifolia); Lavender is a herb recognized for its soothing fragrance, which can be used in forms such, as essential oil diffusers or brewed as herbal tea to help alleviate anxiety.

Skullcap (Scutellaria lateriflora); Skullcap is an herb known for its calming effects, on tension and ability to promote relaxation. It is commonly utilized in tinctures.

St. John's Wort (Hypericum perforatum); St. John's Wort is a remedy with both antidepressant and anxiety reducing properties. It can be beneficial in managing symptoms of mild to moderate anxiety and depression.

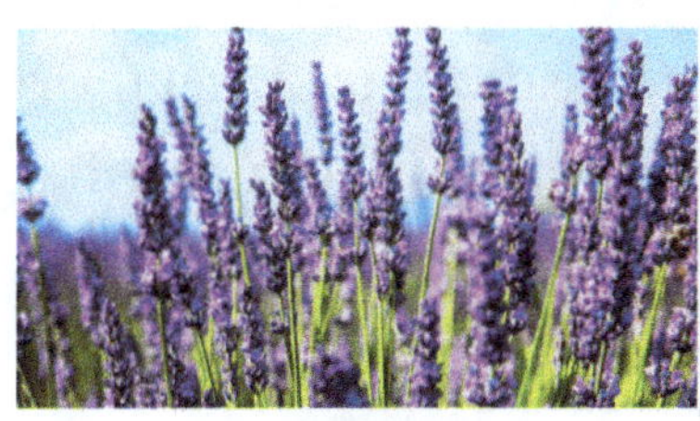

Lavender

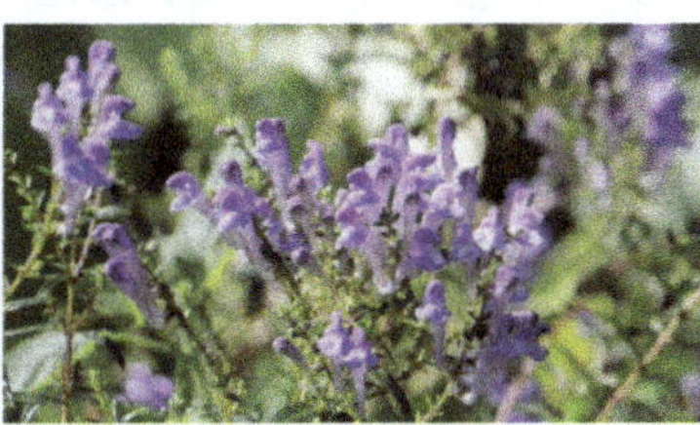

Skullcap

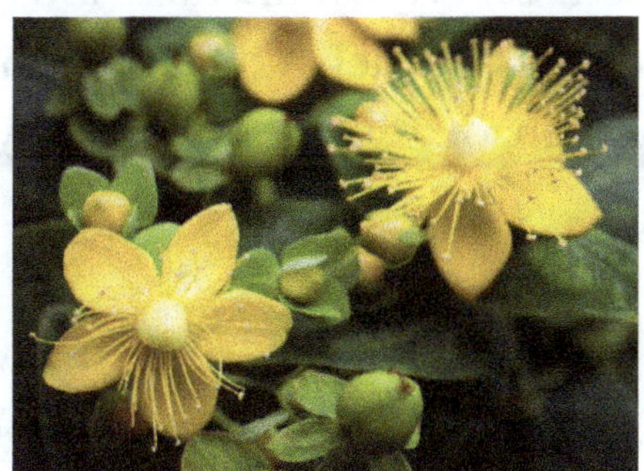

St. John's Wort

Herbal Remedies for Managing Stress and Anxiety

Now that we have explored some categories to address stress and anxiety, let us discuss how to incorporate these herbs into remedies;

Herbal Teas; Many of the previously mentioned herbs can be prepared as soothing herbal teas. Simply steep the dried herbs like Chamomile (Matricaria chamomilla), Lemon Balm (Melissa officinalis), Passionflower (Passiflora incarnata) or Lavender (Lavandula angustifolia) in hot water for 5-10 minutes strain and enjoy. Drink a cup 2-3 times a day whenever necessary before bedtime.

Herbal Tinctures; Herbal tinctures are concentrated extracts derived from herbs. You can. Purchase made tinctures or create your own.

How to Prepare Herbal Tinctures

The process of making tinctures is simple yet effective, in extracting compounds from herbs for diverse purposes.

Here's a simple guide, on how to create your tincture. You'll need the following ingredients;

- Dried or fresh herbs (it's better to use dried herbs as they have moisture)
- Alcohol (common choices include vodka, brandy or rum)
- A glass jar with a lid
- A fine mesh strainer or cheesecloth
- A dark glass bottle, for storing the tincture

Now let's go through the steps;

1. Choose the herb you'd like to use for your tincture.
2. Here are the paraphrased steps, for preparing an infusion;

3. Determine the amount of herbs you'll need. As a rule, use one part dried herbs to five parts alcohol by weight. For example if you have 1 ounce of dried herbs you would need 5 ounces of alcohol.

4. Prepare the herbs by chopping or grinding ones or slightly grinding dried ones to increase their surface area.

5. Take a clean glass jar with a lid and place the prepared herbs inside it. Make sure the jar is clean and dry beforehand.

6. Pour alcohol over the herbs to completely submerge them ensuring they are covered by least an inch or two.

7. Seal the jar tightly with its lid.

8. Give the jar a shake to evenly distribute the alcohol throughout the mixture and then store it in a dark place away, from direct sunlight – like a kitchen cabinet or pantry.

9. Allow the mixture to macerate (soak) for a period of time in order for the flavors to infuse properly.

10. The duration of maceration can differ depending on the herbs used and the desired potency. Typically maceration times fall within the range of 2 to 6 weeks. For instance delicate herbs such, as chamomile may require around 2 weeks whereas stronger herbs, like echinacea might need a period of 4 to 6 weeks.

11. Remember to shake the jar or whenever you remember during the maceration period. This helps in the extraction process.

12. Once the maceration period is finished, strain the mixture by using a fine mesh strainer or cheesecloth into a bowl or another glass jar. Squeeze the herbs to get out liquid as possible.

13. Now transfer the tincture into a glass bottle for proper storage. Remember that dark glass helps protect the tincture from light which can cause degradation of its

compounds. Make sure the bottle has a lid.

14. Take a moment to label the bottle with information such as the herb used, type of alcohol, date of preparation and any other relevant details.

15. Store your tincture in a dark place for preservation. When you want to use it determine a dosage based on your needs and the herbs properties. Usually it's best to take dropperfuls diluted in water or juice.

16. Keep in mind that alcohol-based tinctures have a long shelf life, often lasting for several years. Over time, the tincture may become stronger as more of the herb's properties are extracted.

Chapter Five

Using Herbs, for Natural Pain Relief

Pain is something we all experience at some point in life. That doesn't mean we have to depend on medications from the store or doctors prescriptions, for relief. Mother Nature has blessed us with a variety of herbs that possess the ability to naturally alleviate pain. In this chapter we will delve into the realm of remedies specifically designed to provide relief from pain. We'll explore their mechanisms of action. Learn how to effectively incorporate them into our lives.

Understanding Pain

Pain is a diverse experience that can take on various forms, such, as acute or chronic pain. It acts as a warning system alerting us to harm or injury. However chronic pain, which persists after the initial cause has healed, can have an impact on our overall well-being.

To effectively manage pain it is crucial to have an understanding of its underlying mechanisms. Pain can arise from factors like inflammation, nerve damage, muscle tension or a combination thereof. Herbal remedies offer an approach by targeting these sources of pain and providing relief without the side effects often associated with pharmaceutical pain relievers.

Herbal Pain Relief Mechanisms

Herbs work in ways to alleviate pain naturally. Here are some common mechanisms through which herbs can provide relief;

1. Anti-Inflammatory; Many herbs possess inflammatory properties that help reduce pain caused by inflammation. Turmeric, ginger and boswellia are examples of herbs.

2. Analgesic; Certain herbs have properties that directly relieve pain. Willow bark is one herb that contains compounds similar to aspirin and exerts analgesic effects.

3. Muscle Relaxation; Herbs like valerian and kava kava have muscle relaxing properties that can ease tension related pains, like muscle spasms.

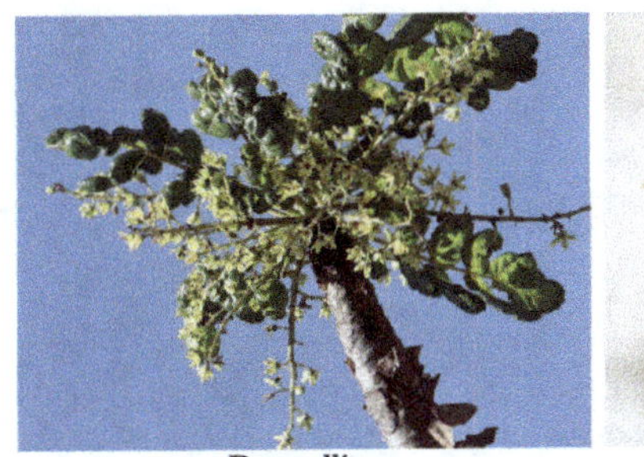

Boswellia

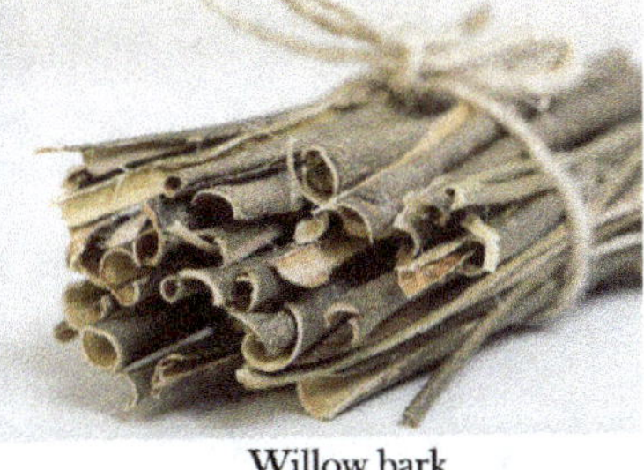

Willow bark

Chapter Six

Herbal Remedies for Digestive Issues

Digestive disorders are a common health issues are a health problem that affects a significant number of people. These problems can range from conditions like indigestion and bloating to more serious conditions such as gastroesophageal reflux disease (GERD) and irritable bowel syndrome (IBS). While conventional medicine offers various treatments for digestive disorders, herbal remedies have been used for centuries to relieve symptoms and promote digestive health. In this chapter we will explore herbs and natural remedies that can effectively address disorders.

Understanding Digestive Conditions

Digestive conditions encompass a variety of disorders that affect the gastrointestinal (GI) tract. Some encountered digestive conditions include;

1. Gastroesophageal Reflux Disease (GERD); GERD is characterized by acid reflux leading to symptoms, like heartburn, regurgitation and irritation of the esophagus.

2. Irritable Bowel Syndrome (IBS); IBS is a disorder of the GI tract with symptoms such as pain, bloating, diarrhea and constipation.

3. Inflammatory Bowel Disease (IBD); IBD includes conditions like Crohns disease and ulcerative colitis that affect the GI tract. Common symptoms include diarrhea, abdominal pain and fatigue.

4. Indigestion (Dyspepsia); Indigestion refers to discomfort or pain in the abdomen often accompanied by bloating, belching and nausea.

5. Constipation; Constipation is characterized by infrequent bowel movements and difficulty passing stools.

6. Diarrhea; Diarrhea involves passage of watery stools and can be caused by various factors such as infections or dietary issues.

Herbal Remedies for Digestive Conditions
Peppermint (Mentha piperita);

Peppermint is well known for its soothing effect on the digestive system. It contains menthol which helps relax the muscles, in the GI tract providing relief from indigestion bloating and abdominal pain.

Drinking peppermint tea or taking peppermint capsules may also have the benefit of soothing the esophageal sphincter which can help decrease the chances of experiencing acid reflux. Peppermint tea or capsules are often utilized to alleviate symptoms associated with bowel syndrome (IBS) and digestive spasms.

Here's how you can prepare peppermint tea; 1-2 teaspoons of dried peppermint leaves, in water for 10-15 minutes. You can sip on this tea before or after meals, for relief.

Peppermint oil capsules are available and can be taken as directed on the product label.

Ginger (Zingiber officinale);

For centuries ginger has been utilized to assist with digestion and provide relief from various digestive disorders. It contains compounds, like gingerol and shogaol which possess inflammatory properties which we had aforementioned in previous chapters and can effectively alleviate symptoms such as nausea, indigestion and bloating. Whether consumed as root in the form of tea or in capsule form ginger aids in promoting digestion and easing gastrointestinal discomfort. Additionally it is beneficial for combating motion sickness.

To create ginger tea slices of ginger in hot water for about 10-15 minutes. Consume it either before or after meals.

Ginger capsules or tablets are readily available and should be taken as directed on the product label.

Chamomile (Matricaria chamomilla);

As mentioned in previous chapters, chamomile is an herb renowned for its calming properties. It effectively soothes the system while reducing inflammation and relieving symptoms of indigestion, gas and bloating. Consuming chamomile tea after meals is a practice to promote relaxation and aid digestion.

To prepare chamomile tea 1-2 teaspoons of dried chamomile flowers in water for approximately 10-15 minutes. Enjoy it before or, after meals.

Fennel (Foeniculum vulgare);

Fennel seeds have long been recognized as a digestive aid.

They contain substances that can relax the muscles, in the tract, which can help reduce symptoms of indigestion, bloating and gas. Having fennel tea or chewing on fennel seeds may provide relief from discomfort. Support healthy digestion.

To prepare fennel tea, steep 1-2 teaspoons of crushed fennel seeds in water for 10-15 minutes. Enjoy it after meals to aid digestion.

Slippery Elm (Ulmus rubra);

Slippery elm is a remedy known for its soothing properties, on the digestive system.

When mixed with water it creates a gel substance that can be beneficial, for coating and protecting the stomach and intestinal lining. This particular herb is commonly used to alleviate symptoms related to acid reflux, gastritis and inflammatory bowel diseases.

To create a soothing gel, simply mix elm powder with water. Drink it as necessary before or after meals.

Licorice (Glycyrrhiza glabra);

Licorice root has a history of use in medicine due to its medicinal properties. It contains compounds that can help reduce inflammation in the tract and promote ulcer healing. Many people find relief from acid reflux, heartburn and stomach ulcers by consuming licorice tea or taking deglycyrrhizinated licorice (DGL) supplements.

To prepare licorice root tea, 1-2 teaspoons of dried licorice root in water for 10-15 minutes. Drink it before or after meals.

For convenience you can also find licorice supplements like deglycyrrhizinated licorice (DGL) tablets that come with dosage instructions on the product label.

Aloe Vera (Aloe barbadensis miller);

Aloe vera has benefits for reducing irritation in the esophagus and providing relief from **GERD** symptoms. Additionally it may help alleviate constipation due, to its effects.

It is advised to consume quantities of aloe vera gel or juice (following the product label) when experiencing symptoms of **GERD** or constipation. However it's important to exercise caution, with aloe vera as consumption may lead to discomfort.

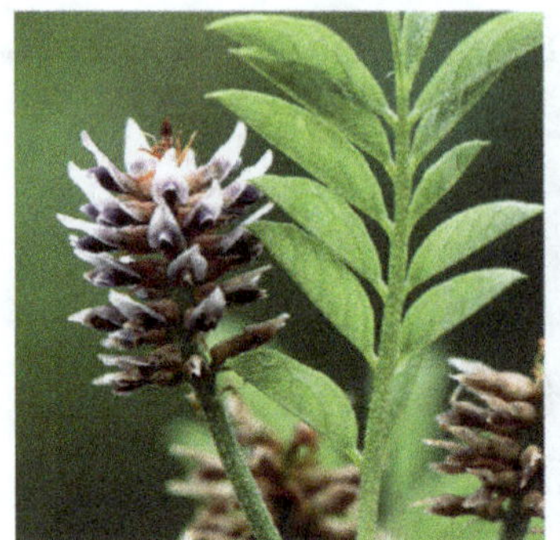

Licorice

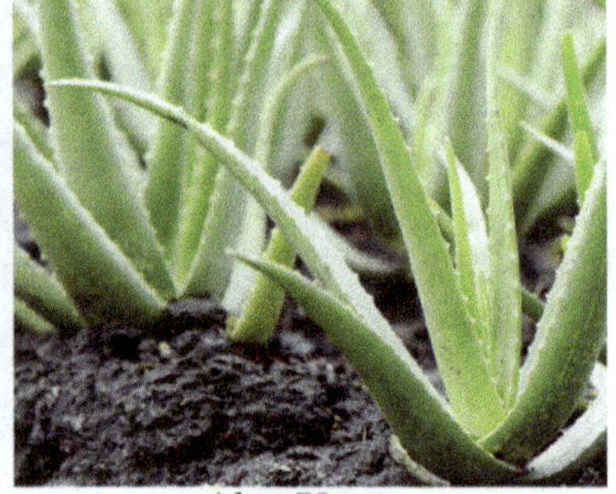

Aloe Vera

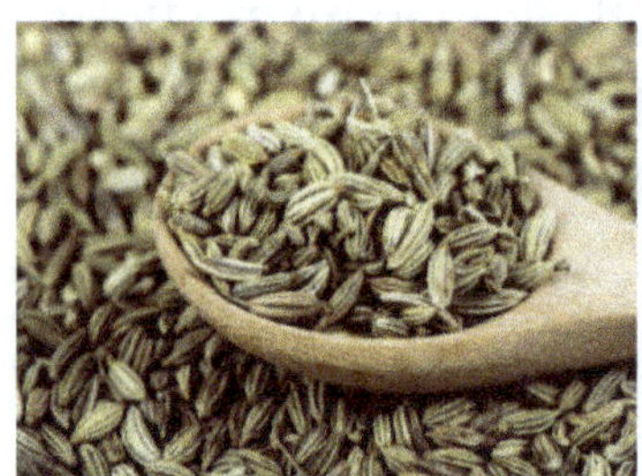

Fennel Seeds

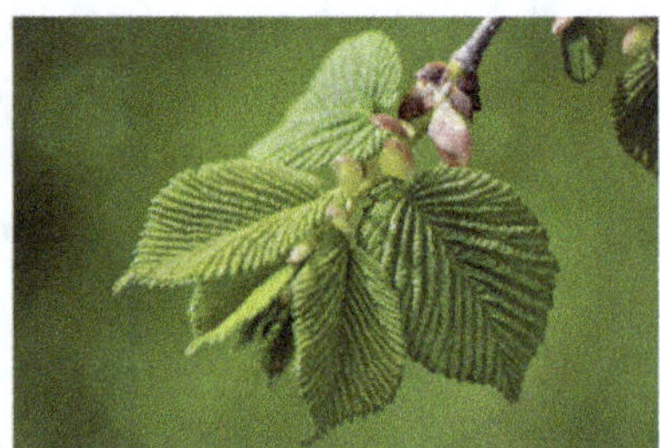

Slippery Elm

Chapter Seven

Enhancing Immune Health Naturally

Having a system is essential, for protecting our bodies against infections, illnesses and diseases. While genetics play a role in our immune health, lifestyle choices and natural remedies can significantly influence the strength of our immune response. In this section we will explore ways to naturally enhance our immunity with a focus on nutrition, lifestyle choices and herbal remedies.

Understanding How the Immune System Works

The system is a network made up of cells, tissues and organs that work together to protect our body from harmful pathogens like bacteria, viruses and fungi. It consists of two components;

1. Innate Immunity; This is the body's line of defense against pathogens. It provides protection that's not specific to any particular pathogen. Physical barriers like the skin and immune cells

such as neutrophils and macrophages are part of this defense mechanism.

2. Adaptive Immunity; This component tailors the body's response to pathogens. It involves producing antibodies and developing immune memory so that if we encounter a pathogen again in the future our immune system can recognize it and fight it off effectively.

The Importance of Nutrition

Maintaining a balanced diet is crucial for supporting an immune system. Various nutrients, vitamins and minerals play roles in boosting function. Here are some key dietary components that contribute to health;

#Vitamin C; Known for its properties that enhance immunity this vitamin can be found abundantly in fruits like oranges and lemons as well, as strawberries and bell peppers.

#Vitamin D plays a role, in regulating our immune system. It can be acquired by spending time in sunlight, consuming fatty fish and opting for dairy products.

#Zinc is vital for the development and proper functioning of our cells. Foods such, as beans, nuts and whole grains are sources of zinc.

#Probiotics; Maintaining a strong immune system is closely tied to having a healthy gut. Probiotic-rich foods like yogurt and kefir can help promote gut health.

#Antioxidants;To safeguard cells from damage caused by radicals it's important to consume antioxidants found in fruits and vegetables.

#Garlic; Garlic contains allicin, which is known for its antimicrobial properties. Incorporating garlic into your meals may assist in preventing infections.

#Turmeric; Turmeric contains curcumin, a compound that has inflammatory and antioxidant effects. These effects can provide support to the immune system.

In addition to following a diet there are lifestyle practices that can contribute to a robust immune system;

1. **Engage in exercise;** Physical activity enhances circulation and facilitates the movement of immune cells throughout the body. Aim for 150 minutes of moderate exercise per week.

2. **Prioritize adequate sleep;** Getting quality sleep is essential for maintaining immunity. Aim for 7-9 hours of sleep each night.

3. **Manage stress;** Chronic stress can weaken the system so it's important to practice stress reduction techniques like meditation, deep breathing or yoga.

4. **Stay hydrated;** Proper hydration supports health and aids in maintaining immune function.

5. **Practice good hand hygiene;** Thoroughly washing your hands helps prevent the spread of infections.

6. **Foster social connections;** Maintaining connections and prioritizing emotional wellbeing can have positive impacts, on immunity.

Boosting the Immune System Naturally

Throughout history herbs have been utilized in medicine as remedies to enhance the immune system. Here are a few solutions that are recognized for their immune boosting properties;

1. Echinacea (Echinacea purpurea); Echinacea is a known herb that supports the system and is commonly used to alleviate the duration and intensity of cold symptoms.

2. Astragalus (Astragalus membranaceus); Astragalus acts as a herb potentially fortifying the system and providing protection, against infections.

3. Elderberry (Sambucus nigra); Elderberry possesses antiviral properties and is commonly used to alleviate the intensity of flu symptoms.

3. Garlic (Allium sativum); Garlic's antimicrobial properties can assist in preventing infections.

4. Medicinal Mushrooms; Reishi, shiitake and maitake mushrooms contain compounds that can support the functioning of the system.

5. Ginger (Zingiber officinale); Ginger has anti-inflammatory and antioxidant effects that may enhance immunity.

6. Turmeric (Curcuma longa); The curcumin found in turmeric has properties that can help regulate the immune system.

Refer to page 26 and 27 for information on how these herbs can be prepared as tea.

Strengthening immunity naturally involves taking an approach that encompasses nutrition, lifestyle choices and herbal remedies. By making decisions about your diet, habits and incorporating supplements wisely you can bolster your immune system and better protect your body against infections and illnesses. It's important to remember that while these strategies can support your health they should not substitute medical advice or treatment when necessary.

Chapter Eight

Herbs for Women's Health

Women's health is a complex aspect of wellbeing that encompasses various stages of life—from puberty and reproductive years to pregnancy, menopause and beyond. Throughout these stages women may face a range of health challenges along, with fluctuations. For years herbal remedies have been widely used to support women's health in a holistic way. In this chapter we will delve into herbs that have traditionally been employed to address women's health issues and enhance overall wellbeing.

The Significance of Herbs, in Women's Health

Throughout centuries herbs have played a part in promoting women's health by providing remedies for a range of health concerns. These plant-based treatments are often selected for their ability to promote hormonal balance, alleviate menstrual discomfort, improve fertility and reduce menopausal symptoms. Let's explore some herbs that can benefit women's health.

1. **Vitex (Chaste Tree Berry);** Restoring Hormonal Balance

Benefits; Vitex, also known as Chaste Tree Berry is a herb frequently recognized as "the women's herb." It has a background, in addressing hormonal imbalances and irregular periods. Vitex aids in regulating the menstrual cycle, easing premenstrual syndrome (PMS) symptoms and enhancing fertility.

Usage; Vitex is commonly consumed in the form of tinctures, capsules or dried berries. For results on balance it is recommended for women to use it consistently for several months.

Vitex acts on the gland to help regulate levels of luteinizing hormone (LH) and follicle-stimulating hormone (FSH). By doing so, it indirectly influences the balance of estrogen and progesterone, helping to normalize the menstrual cycle.

2. Black Cohosh; Alleviating Menopausal Symptoms

Benefits; Black Cohosh is a herbal remedy, for women who experience discomfort during menopause. It works really well in reducing hot flashes, mood swings, sleep troubles and vaginal dryness that often come with menopause. You can usually take Black Cohosh as a tincture or, in capsules. It might take few weeks of using it to *notice improvements in menopausal symptoms.*

Usage; Black Cohosh has compounds that interact with serotonin receptors in the brain. This interaction may assist in regulating body temperature and mood. That's why it's considered an herb for women going through the transition of menopause.

3. Red Raspberry Leaf; Supporting Uterine Health

Benefits; Red Raspberry Leaf is a tonic that promotes women's wellbeing, during different stages of life. It helps strengthen the uterus, cramps, improve fertility and prepare the body for childbirth.

Usage; Red Raspberry Leaf is commonly consumed as a nourishing tea. It can be enjoyed daily throughout the cycle. It is particularly recommended during pregnancy to support uterine health.

Red Raspberry Leaf is packed with nutrients such as vitamins C and B, calcium, iron and magnesium. These nutrients contribute to its ability to tone the uterine muscles and provide relief from discomfort. During pregnancy it can aid in preparing the uterus for labor.

4. Dong Quai; Balancing Hormones

Benefits; Dong Quai, often known as "ginseng " holds a place in traditional Chinese medicine. It helps regulate cycles, ease menstrual cramps and promote hormonal balance.

Usage; Dong Quai comes in forms including tinctures, capsules or dried root, for making tea. It's advisable to consult with a healthcare professional regarding dosage and usage instructions.

Dong Quai contains compounds called coumarins which are known to have mild estrogenic effects.

These substances have the potential to regulate hormone levels, in women, which can be especially beneficial for individuals with cycles or who experience premenstrual syndrome (PMS).

5. Maca; Improving Fertility and Sexual Desire

Benefits; Maca is a type of adaptogenic herb that has become popular due to its ability to promote hormonal equilibrium, elevate energy levels and enhance sexual desire. It is commonly utilized by women seeking to improve their fertility and overall sexual wellbeing.

Usage: You can incorporate maca powder into your diet by adding it to smoothies, beverages or food. It is advisable to start with a small amount and gradually increase the dosage as needed. Maca contains glucosinolates which have the ability to influence the endocrine system helping to balance hormones. This herb is highly regarded for its potential to enhance libido and overall vitality.

6. **Wild Yam:** Menopausal Relief

Benefits: For relief from symptoms such as hot flashes, mood swings and vaginal dryness, wild yam is commonly used. It can also help regulate fluctuations during menopause.

Usage: Wild yam is available in forms including tinctures, capsules and topical creams that are applied to the skin for absorption. The compound diosgenin found in yam can be converted into progesterone in the body potentially alleviating symptoms associated with declining hormone levels.

7. **Shatavari:** Balancing Hormones and Supporting Fertility

Benefits: Shatavari is a herb renowned for its rejuvenating properties and ability to balance hormones. It supports women's health, enhances fertility and aids lactation.

Usage: Shatavari can be consumed daily in powder form, capsules or tinctures to promote wellbeing.

Shatavari has compounds that function, as phytoestrogens, which're capable of aiding in the regulation of hormone levels in women. It is a herb known for its ability to promote balance and support fertility.

8. **Nettle:** Nutrient-Rich Support

Benefits: Nettle is a nutrient-rich herb that can help alleviate symptoms of **PMS** and menopause. It serves as a source of vitamins and minerals that contribute to health.

Usage: Nettle can be enjoyed as a nourishing herbal tea or Incorporated into your diet as a leafy green vegetable. It is generally considered safe for consumption.

Nettle is packed with vitamins such as **A, C** and **K** along with minerals like calcium, magnesium and iron. These beneficial nutrients make it an excellent addition to the diet for women who want to address nutritional deficiencies and enhance their wellbeing.

9. **Licorice Root:** Hormone Balance

Licorice root is beneficial in maintaining hormone balance alleviating symptoms of **PMS** and supporting adrenal health. It has properties that can provide relief from menstrual discomfort.

Usage: You can find licorice root in forms such as tinctures, capsules or teas. It's important to use it in moderation and seek guidance from a healthcare professional if you have high blood pressure.

Licorice root contains glycyrrhizin, which has the ability to mimic cortisols effects in the body. This quality helps maintain adrenal function and hormonal equilibrium in women.

10. **Motherwort:** Calming and Uterine-Toning

Motherwort is renowned for its calming effects on the body and its ability to tone the uterus. It can assist in relieving menstrual cramps and anxiety while promoting heart health.

Usage: Typically consumed as a tincture, motherwort offers calming benefits for women seeking relaxation and uterine support. You can take it as needed to alleviate menstrual discomfort or reduce stress.

Motherwort contains compounds that aid in relaxing the muscles of the uterus thereby easing menstrual cramps. Moreover its calming properties can offer relief from anxiety and stress which can worsen symptoms associated with PMS.

Recommendation: *For Hormonal related issues and endometriosis, I strongly recommend a book titled "Healing: How I Overcame Endometriosis" authored by Susan J. Derek.*

You can look it up on amazon.com

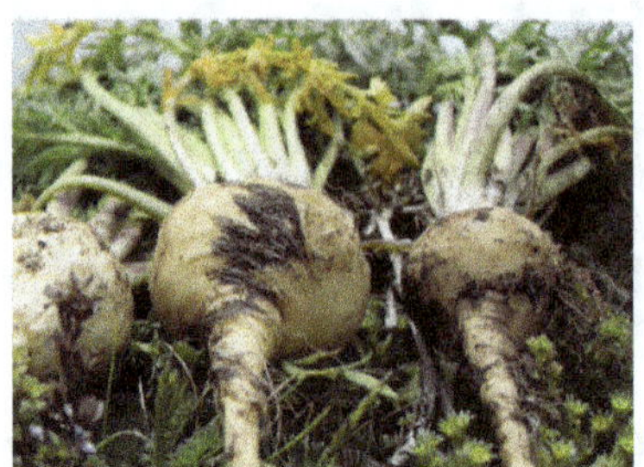

Maca

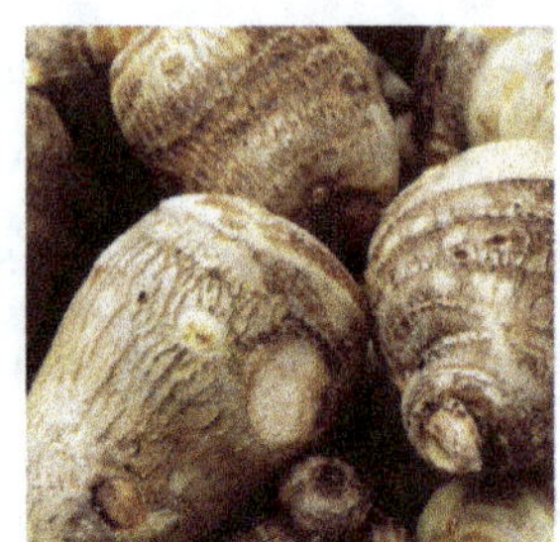

Wild Yam

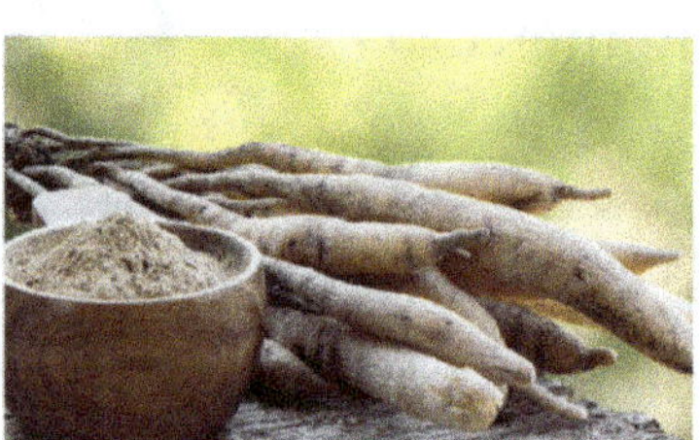

Shatavari

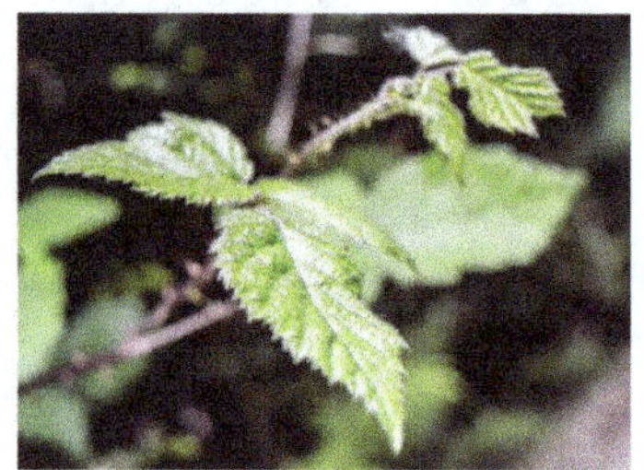

Nettle

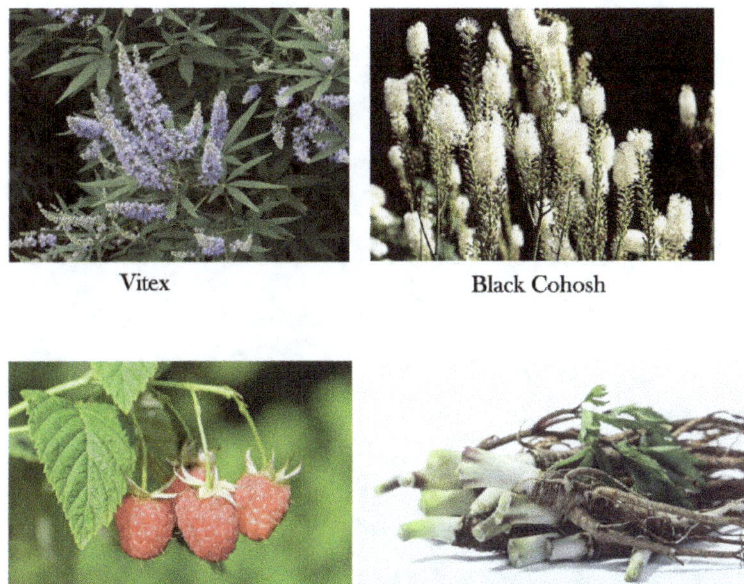

Vitex

Black Cohosh

Red Raspberry Leaf

Dong Quai Root

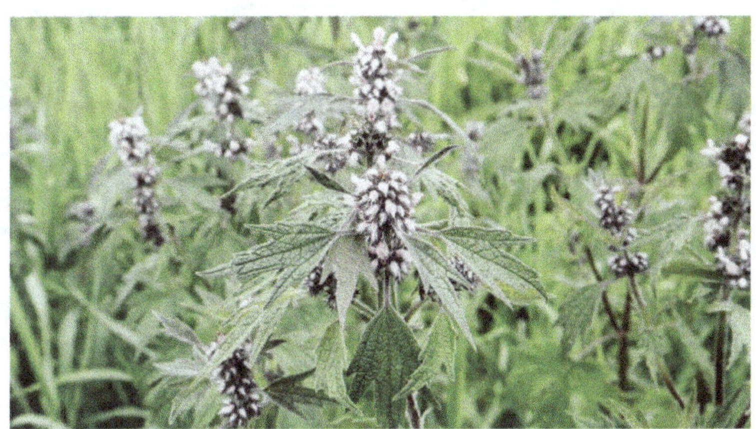

Motherwort

Chapter Nine

Natural Herbal Treatments, for Children

The wellbeing and health of our children are of importance to us as parents and caregivers. We often look for natural safe methods to support their health. For generations, herbal remedies have been used to address childhood ailments and discomforts. In this chapter we will delve into the realm of treatments for children focusing on practices common issues faced during childhood and effective herbal solutions.

Ensuring the Safety of Herbal Remedies for Children

Before we explore specific herbal remedies, it is vital to address the safety concerns associated with using herbs for children. While herbs can provide effective solutions they must be used cautiously under the guidance of a healthcare professional. Here are some important safety considerations;

Dosages Appropriate for Age; When administering remedies to children it is crucial to adjust the dosages based on their age and weight. Infants and young children generally require lower doses compared to children.

Consulting a Healthcare Professional; It is always advisable to consult with a healthcare provider like a professional herbalist before giving herbal remedies to children, babies and infants. They can offer guidance on dosages well as potential interactions with medications.

Emphasizing Quality; Opt for quality herbs from reputable sources, in order to ensure purity and potency.

When selecting herbs it's important to steer of any that may have come into contact, with pesticides or harmful substances. Remember that children can have sensitivities to herbs so it's advisable to start with amounts and observe how

they respond. If any negative reactions occur it's
best to stop using the herbs.

Additionally there are herbs that are not
recommended for babies and infants. Examples
of herbs include eucalyptus and specific types of
herbal teas like Peppermint (Mentha piperita),
Licorice (Glycyrrhiza glabra), Licorice
(Glycyrrhiza glabra), Saw Palmetto (Serenoa
repens), Black Cohosh (Actaea racemosa),
Aconite (Aconitum napellus), Wormwood
(Artemisia absinthium), Pennyroyal (Mentha
pulegium) and Yohimbe (Pausinystalia yohimbe).
Always check the safety of specific herbs before
use.

Gradual Introduction; Gradually introduce herbs
to observe how your child reacts. This will help
you identify any allergies or sensitivities they may
have.

Common Childhood Ailments and Herbal Solutions

Now let's explore some health issues that
children often experience and the herbal

remedies that can provide relief while promoting wellbeing.

1. Digestive Discomfort;

Common Issues; Children frequently experience discomfort such, as colic, gas, indigestion and constipation.

Herbal Solutions;

Fennel (Foeniculum vulgare); You can use fennel tea or glycerite to alleviate gas and colic in infants and young children.

Chamomile (Matricaria chamomilla); Chamomile tea is soothing and can relieve indigestion, colic and promote relaxation.

Ginger (Zingiber officinale); For older children, ginger tea or ginger chews can be helpful for nausea and upset stomach.

2. Cough and Cold;

Common Issues; Childhood is often plagued by coughs, colds and congestion.

Herbal Solutions;

Honey; If your child's over one year old, honey can soothe coughs and sore throats. Simply mix a teaspoon with water or herbal tea.

Elderberry (Sambucus nigra); Known for its immune boosting properties elderberry syrup can help shorten the duration of colds.

Thyme (Thymus vulgaris); You can use thyme tea or thym- infused honey to relieve coughs and congestion.

Eucalyptus (Eucalyptus globulus); When children are older than two years, taking a steam bath infused with eucalyptus can assist in relieving congestion.

3. Teething Discomfort;

Common Challenges; Teething can be a period for both babies and parents due, to the discomfort. Irritability it brings.

Herbal Remedies;

Chamomile (Matricaria chamomilla); Chamomile tea can be used to soothe teething pain. Simply dip a cloth in chamomile tea freeze it and allow the baby to chew on it.

Catnip (Nepeta cataria); Catnip tea is another option that can help alleviate teething discomfort in infants.

Cloves: Clove oil, diluted in carrier oil and applied topically to the gums, can provide relief. It's important to ensure that the clove oil is properly diluted to avoid any irritation.

4. Skin Irritations;

Common Problems; Children often experience skin irritations, like diaper rash, eczema and insect bites.

Natural Remedies;

Calendula (Calendula officinalis); Applying calendula cream or oil directly on the area can help soothe diaper rash and minor skin irritations.

Chamomile (Matricaria chamomilla); Using chamomile-infused cream or oil can provide relief for eczema and irritated skin.

Lavender (Lavandula angustifolia); Diluted lavender essential oil mixed with carrier oil can alleviate discomfort caused by insect bites while promoting relaxation.

5. Sleep Issues;

Common Problems; Sleep difficulties can affect children of all ages.

Natural Remedies;

Lavender (Lavandula angustifolia); Placing a drops of lavender essential oil in a diffuser or applying it to bedding before bedtime can encourage relaxation and improve sleep quality.

Chamomile (Matricaria chamomilla); Offering chamomile tea before bedtime can have a soothing effect.

Valerian (Valeriana officinalis); For children, with sleep issues valerian root may be used under the guidance of a healthcare professional.

6. Fever and Pain;

Common Problems; Fever and pain are frequently experienced by children often due to minor illnesses.

Herbal Remedies;

Willow Bark (Salix spp.); Willow bark, similar to aspirin is a source of salicin. It can be used with guidance to alleviate pain in older children.

Echinacea (Echinacea purpurea); Echinacea can assist in boosting the system during times of illness.

7. Stress and Anxiety;

Common Problems; Children might experience stress and anxiety due to reasons such as school, social situations or changes in their environment.

Herbal Remedies;

Chamomile (Matricaria chamomilla); Drinking chamomile tea can help induce a sense of calmness and reduce anxiety feelings.

Lemon Balm (Melissa officinalis); Consuming lemon balm tea or tincture can aid in relaxation. Alleviate nervousness.

Passionflower (Passiflora incarnata); With guidance, passionflower can be used to address anxiety and restlessness in children.

8. Attention and Focus;

Common Problems; Some children may face challenges when it comes to attention and focus which can affect their learning abilities and behavior.

Herbal Remedies;

Ginkgo (Ginkgo biloba); Ginkgo leaf extract may assist in cognitive function and attention enhancement for older children.

Gotu Kola (Centella asiatica); Gotu kola is known to support clarity and improve focus, in children.